THE 4 PAINFUL LIFE STORIES

HOW WE CONTRACTED HIV/AIDS

Special Dedication

To anyone infected with the hiv/aids, there is always light at the end of the tunnel.

Acknowledgements

I am most appreciative of the many people who offered their invaluable views, ideas and support towards the making of this book.

In particular, I want to thank, with lots of humility, my family and close friends for those relentless prayers and support without which, I doubt if this material would have seen light of the day. Thank you all and may God the Almighty bless you richly.

Finally, but most important, I thank God for the gift of life and for His endless blessings upon my life. Indeed, great His faithfulness. His grace, love and mercy endure forever!

Contents

Always Look Around

I once had no food to eat, until I met a man who had no teeth!

I once had no good shoes to wear, until I met a man who had no feet!

I once had no nice shirt to wear, until I met a man who had no arms!

I once had no money, until I met a dead beggar on a busy street!

Anonymous

When your life is on a downhill and you seem to be totally defeated, don't ever give up. Out there, someone else has it even worse. When you look around, you'll be glad yours isn't that worse! Your life could only seem like an endless curse only if you shut yourself in your own world, refusing to look around.

Always Look Around

Finish everyday and be done with it. You have done what you could. Some blunders and absurdities, no doubt crept in. Forget them as soon as you can. Tomorrow is a new day. Begin it well. Do not let your old nonsense destroy such a new day

Ralph Waldo Emerson.

The Big Question

Life can at times turn out to be mean, if not cruel! Many of us dream of being in possession of the beautiful things this life can offer, yet in the process, forget that even the beautiful of roses have thorns. What would you do when life confronts you with its ugly side and in a flash, scatters all of your dreams?

This book in a nutshell

Herein are touching accounts of Angela, James, Elizabeth and Anne, four innocent characters who were unknowingly, each infected with the aids causing virus.

Each of their detailed moving stories are not only heart-breaking to read through, but are equally thought-provoking and packed with life-changing wisdom. Their unique predicaments eye-opens the reader to the reality that we are all, at any given time, in danger of hiv infection. And sometimes, the infection can occur in the most unlikely of places - like in a bloody road accident; read Anne's miserable story. No one is therefore safe!

The resolve of the four characters and commitment to individually carry their own respective crosses, in broad daylight, however heavy the crosses seem, is a real wake-up call for everyone to embrace and unreservedly support persons infected with HIV. After all, even if you may not be directly infected with the virus, you are still affected, directly or indirectly: that infected person may be your relative, a friend, colleague, fellow citizen, and most significant, a fellow human being.

So many people infected with hiv have over the years retreated to a silent world and helplessly watched their self-esteem go up in smoke, so fast, due to stigma. They simply cannot stomach being seen as 'infected' and therefore, live in constant worry of what other people might be thinking or saying about them.

Angela, James, Elizabeth, and Anne are four phony characters with life-changing fables about how they were each caught up in the hiv/aids trap. Their stories not only motivate, but also offer encouragement to the rest of *their society*; those infected with the virus, to keep fighting on with boldness to experience the beauty of the next day, tomorrow. The stories herein offer an almost tangible encouragement to any hiv-positive person not to lose focus or hope in life simply because of a mere ailment.

Still, the heart-wrenching narrations encourages the rest of the world never to discriminate anyone on the basis of their hiv status. Not until you put on another's shoes, you may never know how far you can walk in them.

This read further outlines some outstanding and realistic reasons as to why anyone should never attempt to commit suicide, regardless of any ugly life's predicament. It also details the six most common notorious beliefs and misconceptions about sex and hiv/aids. And in its finality, it presents the reader with an opportunity to understand some of the reasons as to why God may allow someone to go through an unexplainably strange and difficult ordeal.

Knowing that you are allocating your most precious resource, time, to go through this material, I am more than humbled and wish to assure you reading this book to its end is one invaluable investment you'll forever cherish taking. **And most importantly the author has done all these for the sake of charity!**

Welcome and let's begin the journey.

The Build Up

A journey of a thousand miles begins with a single step

Lao Tzu

The cloudy afternoon of Saturday 26th November, 2011 is in Juma's memory as a life changing and eye-opening day. That fateful afternoon, he was out with a group of colleagues for an annual corporate social responsibility activity at a local health center. The facility was located a few blocks away from Juma's company's head office.

Whenever they had such events, they had a tradition of donating select personal effects and foodstuff. On that day, they had carried seven cartons of laundry detergents and twelve boxes filled with an assortment of foodstuff, all of which they were excited to donate to the facility.

By 3.00 pm, they made their way into the facility and were heartily welcomed by Dr. Robert, the institution's administrator who was anxiously awaiting their arrival. Very warm, charming, and jovial are lesser adjectives in describing how happy Dr. Robert appeared while receiving the guests. Without hesitation, he ushered them into his neatly arranged and spacious office.

On that day, members supported by the facility had a group bonding session taking place in the main hall. These members were a small group of persons infected with hiv/aids. Remarkably, they possessed a strong resolve to live the rest of their lives positively. They had a core mission to encourage and support each another, whilst trumpeting to the rest of the world that hiv/aids could possibly infect anyone, anywhere, and at any given time, and that it wasn't a death sentence.

After a few exchanges, Juma and his team were thereafter ushered into the main hall for an occasion that would later on, turn out to be the genesis of the four painful life stories. Once inside the hall, formal introductions preceded an interlude of song performance from the group. Even members of the visiting party were not left behind; they all enthusiastically joined the stage that was fast growing dusty by each passing minute to dance to one famous local celebratory song.

Afterwards, Cleopatra, the group's chairlady, brought forward three women and one gentleman in their late twenties, who one after another, gave moving accounts about how each unknowingly, got infected with the aids causing virus. It is the stories from these four people, as narrated to Juma and his team, which builds up the 4 painful life stories.

Get yourself ready and welcome to **The 4 Painful Life Stories.**

My Sweet College Boyfriend

An emotional episode of Angela, A young female college student who got infected with hiv by her college boyfriend

In the race of life, you can never outpace your shadow by any meaningful distance

F. Otieno

First on stage was Angela, a young female student who got infected with the virus through her college boyfriend.

In a very low but firm voice, she greeted the audience.

"Good evening everyone"

"Good evening"…the audience answered back.

She then went on.

"My name is Angela. I am an only child, and must confess I had a wonderful, secure and happy childhood. I grew up an archetypal spoilt brat, everything I wanted I had. We were a happy family, always jovial and united in love. However, one month after joining college, my parents had an irreconcilable difference. Regrettably, they had to part ways".

She then paused for a moment to catch breath and adjust her now waning tone.

"Ooh sorry girl" … a voice echoed from the audience.

"thank you.", she responded in a more refreshed and clearer tone, and went on.

"Upon completing my first semester studies, I returned home to a gloomy reception by my dad. Hastily, I asked him where mum had gone to. Shockingly, he at first ignored my question. The look and expression on his face was that of *why should I bother to know where she is'*. I didn't suspect that anything unusual could have transpired.

Ignorantly, I again asked him the same question, this time looking straight into his eyes. With lots of hesitation, he mumbled to himself a few words and thereafter, informed me mum had left home for good. At first, I thought I was in some deep dream and had to speedily wake up. I punched myself several times in the arm just to affirm I wasn't in a strange dreamland where I was no longer going to see my mum ever. Sadly, I wasn't dreaming. I was a wake, and everything was real.

To date, I still hear echoes of the painful words my daddy had fumbled close to my ears on that fateful day; *'Your mother is gone forever. She'll probably never return'*. These words made me numb and speechless. For a moment, I thought he was just teasing me, only to feel numb at the weight of his words when reality finally downed on me. Yes, the mighty Babylon had fallen. After all those beautifully fun-filled years, our once happy family was no more.

I wildly ran into my room, locked myself up and cried a river. Uncontrolled tears that freely flew from my eyes ended up wetting my bedding. *What did mummy do that my now strange-behaving dad could not find a heart to forgive?'* I still ask myself even to date!

I later on learnt she had left for overseas to stay with her eldest sister in America. The exact reason as to why they decided to part ways is still a mystery to me. Maybe, it's only time that will tell, some day!

I resumed my second semester studies feeling so low. I felt de-motivated on continued thought of my mothers' absence from home, and from my life. I needed someone to support and console me, but had no one close to confine my issues to. Never in my wildest dreams did I think such division could ever pay our home a visit. Sadly, there it was, a strange reality I had to confront, embrace and live with, probably for the rest of my life! I lonely thought so, most of the time.

I met Joseph, my late college boyfriend one Sunday afternoon as I was out doing some laundry. I instantly liked him not only because of his brave approach, but he was equally charming and befitting the true definition of a handsome young guy. Yes, Joseph was just too sweet for me to ignore his presence and even his pursuit for a relationship. He was every girl's favorite man.

He came into my life at my weakest point. I badly needed someone to heap my fragile fears on. We became instant friends. His friendship and love rejuvenated lost radiance in my life. I somehow felt I had a secure shoulder to lean on. And on each passing day, I found more reasons to love him even more. He was all over my mind and felt closer than my only family, my dad. I stupidly trusted Joseph and shared with him my all. After all, I was a girl in deep love.

On the last week of the second semester, there was an all-night party organized for final year students. Since Joseph too was in his final year of study, he had to be present at that party. That evening, I accompanied him to the graduation square, the party's venue.

Goodness, I had a moment of my life. He warmly held me close to his chest and guided my steps to the rhythms of tunes which were interchangeably playing at very fast, fast, medium, slow and sometimes slower bits.

After several hours of dancing we stopped and proceeded to a nearby tent which had been set up at the corner of the graduation square. It was there where alcoholic drinks were being served. While there, Joseph offered me a bottle of some sweet wine. I can't even recall its label. In my entire life before, I had never taken wine or any other alcoholic drink. Out of love, I obliged and took several gulps straight from the bottle. My goodness, it was so tender and sweet! To his surprise, I drank half the bottle before losing my cool.

Upon realizing I was drunk, Joseph took me to the men's' hostel where I ended up spending the rest of the night in his room, on his bed, with him. That was the fateful night we had an unprotected sex. Equally, it was the night I lost my girlhood.

The next day, I woke up feeling pain all over my body. However, I felt no remorse. I was ready to break any wall anywhere in the world just to prove my love and commitment to Joseph. Yes, I did honestly love him.

When I reported for the second year, I started feeling weak, most of the time. I could easily fall asleep in lecture halls out of unexplained tiredness. The tiredness took a toll on me and I carried it everywhere I went.

One evening, I decided to go for a checkup at the college's health centre. After a thorough blood and body examination, the nurse referred me to the students' counselor, with some sealed envelope. I didn't expect anything big could be the matter. After a few minutes' walk across the lawn, I arrived at the student counselors' office. Actually, it was a three minute walk to be precise.

Fortunately, Mrs. Mulinge, the students' Counselor was in office, all alone and free to attend to me. After greeting her, I innocently handed over to her the sealed envelope, and patiently sat back to a seat she had offered me. Honestly, I inwardly jokingly wondered why I was being referred from a health facility to an office filled with students' files for an interpretation of a medical report! After opening the envelope and going through a note inside, she took a moment of deep silence. Thereafter, she remorsefully looked at me straight in the eyes and inquired about my past relations and sex life. Openly, I told her everything about my Joseph.

She then went into another silent mode, only to resurrect with words which eventually turned my world upside down. As careful as she could, she informed me *'you have an hiv infection'*.

Those words literally, electrocuted my mind. For a moment, I was dead in my thought. It was extremely unbelievable to accept the strange reality that my sweet Joseph could turn out to be such a monster and infect me with the aids causing virus! With lots of regret, I tearfully recalled the unfortunate events of that fateful night. I could not stop blaming myself for letting it happen.

The students' counselor waited with lots of patience, as unending tears of terror and regret freely flowed from my now blurry eyes. I was all alone and bankrupt of words. With lots of unending struggle, she consoled and told me to worry not.

Truth is I was in no position to reverse my condition. I had to fast accept that horrible predicament and move on. I had never had sex before with anyone, and I innocently thought that Joseph too had never had sex before. Shockingly, I was dreadfully wrong! Awfulness, despair and misery engulfed my world. In the course of our relationship, we talked lots of things with Joseph, but we never ever talked about hiv/aids.

We never communicated with Joseph thereafter. On my third year of studies, I overheard he had succumbed to the illness and died at their rural home.

If he knew that he was infected with the virus, why wasn't he on antiretroviral drugs?'…why didn't he tell me? I asked myself severally. Then I recalled how egocentric Joseph was. He was the type of man who could bare-handedly go after a lion all alone in the forest. In my heart, I wanted to forgive him but deep down, my soul just couldn't. *Did he ever feel gratified by poisoning my dignity and self respect?* I opened my heart and loved him like a fool. However, he instead took the burning love I hotly offered and used it to burn down my world!

I feel my life is now meaningless. I struggle to focus on the gloomy future; *a stunning career, a happy new family, beautiful children,* but I wake up each moment to realize I am always in a deep dream. Sometimes I wish I was forever locked in such dreamland.

For sure, I know nothing can stop me from being anything I want to be in the future, but it could have been much better if I were not infected with this virus.

I know I have fallen down, but I will not remain on the ground. I will keep my head high and pray to the Almighty on each passing day to give me the necessary strength and resilience to fight for the invaluable beauty which is embedded in each passing day. Back then I didn't know but know I know that to love is to risk. Access the risk involved before loving anyone deeply.

I believe in the adage *what you don't know might kill you.* When you love someone, get to know about their hiv status.

When was the last time you talked about Hiv/aids with your partner?..............

Don't gamble with your lives. The reality of living on borrowed time is always uncomfortable. Stay safe and enjoy life."

At the Barbershop

When misfortune visited the Barber's

Never take anything for granted

Anonymous

Misfortune is always an un-invited guest. It's restless and often knocks door after door. At times, it forcefully enters some houses, just like an armed robber. Misfortune maybe present even in the most unlikely of places…. began James.

He was second to speak after Angela.

"That Wednesday evening, I left office in a hurry. I wanted to arrive home early that day. I worked as a supervisor in a down town electronic shop, and most of the time, I was used to leaving for home at around at 9.00 pm, everyday. Upon reaching the bus station, the fast growing queue was already long. I figured from where I was to line up, it could roughly take me an hour before boarding the next bus. Readily, I gave up, instead opting to find another creative way of letting time pass by to allow the seemingly still queue cut down its length.

Then the idea of having my hair cut came into my mind, and without hesitation, I checked in at one of the local barbershops, which was adjacent to the bus stage. It was around 6.30 pm, yes, I can still recall vividly.

Weirdly, immediately I made my way inside the barber's, power went off! Was it bad luck? There was a sudden widespread power failure within the town affecting several buildings, including the one housing the barber shop. Unfortunately, that building had no alternative source of power. Since it was getting dark, the Barber simply lit some two candles and continued shaving a gentleman whom he had been shaving before the power went off.

Interestingly, this time round, he substituted his electric enabled hair cutting machine with some hand held hair cutting monster; a gadget that had some attachments of sharp blades on its front end. Sitting on a waiting bench close to the barber, I was both dazzled and scared at how the gadget functioned. I almost gave up, but was quickly re-assured by the Barber the gadget was in perfect condition and functioned even more efficiently than an average electric-enabled haircutting machine. I then patiently waited for my turn to come. However, deep inside, I silently prayed for electric power to resume for my hair to be done with an electric-enabled machine.

Moments later, it was my turn. The Barber hurriedly jumped on my hair without properly sterilizing that monster gadget. I opted to remain silent, never questioning that weird and unprofessional conduct. Anyway, I trusted him and equally thought there was no danger involved. After all, he ended up doing a perfect job on my head.

However, since the room was dimly lit, he ended up making some tiny cuts on my head, which slightly bled thereafter. Due to those tiny cuts, I left the shop with my head itching all over. It was right inside that barbershop, through those cuts that I ended up contracting the deadly aids causing virus.

Truth is I have never stopped blaming myself for that unfortunate incidence. Probably, I should have walked away immediately electric power went off! But unfortunately, there I was, as docile as a cow being led to slaughter house. Sad still, I had insufficient legal grounds to sue the Barber since I didn't have any witness to prove before any judge that my infection came from the barber!

It was after carefully and deeply revisiting my active sex life for the past one year that I authoritatively concluded my infection came on that day of the blackout, at the barber's. I had been going for full body health checkups every six months for the past four years, and apart from some minor ailments, I had been declared hiv-free all along. I equally didn't have anyone close to call my love, and hadn't slept with any lady in over two years. I did all the thoughts and mathematics of how I could have ended up contracting the virus only to be left with that evening at the barber as the only day I could have exposed myself within the six months before going for checkup.

I made a billion dollar mistake that fateful day. Nonetheless, that was my fate and couldn't run way from it. I had to embrace that depressing reality and live with it for the rest of my life!

Since then, I have always had one gospel to spread, especially to men and women who visit barbershops for haircuts: *While visiting any barbershop for haircut, ensure any machine or tool getting into contact with your head or any part of your body is clean and properly sterilized before use.*

We only have one life to live. No one should waste it out of sheer and blatant ignorance. Please don't make the mistake I made. It is tiring to survive each day on drugs. Let's help in the war against hiv/aids and be each other's keepers".

That Night, At the Club

The young lady who got infected with hiv by a stranger, in a local club's gents

Real men date sober women, they don't take advantage of drunken ladies

Francis O

Immediately James left the stage, Elizabeth, one of the three ladies, took over and started a shocking and unbelievably strange narration about how an unfamiliar person infected her with the aids causing virus.

"That Thursday evening, club Ozone was full to its capacity" She cheerfully began, and went on.

"But how did I find myself in club Ozone in the first place?" She paused, then went on. "Here is how…

Being late in the evening and nearing end of the year, several working cadre and students were already off work and classes respectively, justifying the reason for the big, noisy and full of life merrymaking party inside club Ozone. As usual, the disk jockey was on top of his game, playing non-stop rock, my all time favorite music.

That day, I had a bad day at work. My boss felt I had become a thorn in her flesh. She felt I undermined her and that I was fond of treating her as some junior employee within the office. She therefore decided to confront and possibly *put me where I belonged to.*

The scene was nasty and ugly. She shouted at me in full glare of clients and fellow staff. I felt belittled and humiliated. *Has our girlie issues reached this nasty level?*, I inwardly wondered! Anyway, I wasn't all that special. I was just a two-year-old employee, though very ambitious. Well, I didn't believe in *too much ambition can kill someone*. And I still don't. I decided to bite the bullet. I never shouted back. Instead, I retained my calm, though inwardly frustrated, till end of the day. That was why when evening approached, I decided pass by club Ozone to vent off that day's anger and frustration.

I went and sat all alone at the edge of the front counter. Then one by one, I ordered for a few shots of tequila, my favorite drink. I guess I took five shots and afterwards, took to the dance floor. That evening, I was credited with inventing several weird dance styles. The more I danced, the dizzier I felt. The drink was slowly taking a toll on me. I was gradually losing my balance. Hesitantly, I staggered to the washroom.

Time had gone and many revelers had started leaving the club for home.

I still don't know how I ended up in the men's' washroom! Sadly, while there, I lost my balance and fell on the floor. Then out of nowhere, *a drunken Samaritan* came to my rescue. Weirdly, this drunk guy later on turned into *a Mr. quickie*!

As I was uselessly lying down on the gents' floor, I blurrily remember the drunken Samaritan had offered to help lift me up. That day, I had skimpily dressed and my blue inner sexy pants showed off as this mysterious guy lifted me up. I can't clearly recollect what transpired next. However, locked inside one of the toilets, we had a quick one ......gosh! ... it was unprotected!

I had never met this guy in my life before. That was my very first time, nasty and ugly meeting. Everything happened so fast, since other drunken men were now pilling and ruthlessly knocking at the toilet's door which he had locked from the inside.

I regained some sense and braved my way back to my seat. I afterwards cleared my pending bill and called for a taxi home.

I regretted everything the next day. The reality of having unprotected sex eventually hit me. Worse still, I had the unprotected sex with a total stranger! Stupidly, I decided to hide my bizarre ordeal, never telling anyone. I equally never bothered to seek for medical attention. Probably that would have saved me from infection. However, I somehow felt gratified since I had been badly humiliated at work the previous day. That was indeed a weird way to satisfy my already dented ego.

Three months later, I started feeling weak and tired, morning to evening. Sleeping a lot during the day and night became my new norm. However, it's the missing of my monthly girl experience on three consecutive months that finally prompted me to go for a medical checkup.

On a fine Sunday afternoon, I gathered courage and went for check up. Little did I know the unfortunate event at club Ozone would later on haunt me forever! Yes, my blood count had significantly dropped and was confirmed hiv-positive. Equally, I was already three months pregnant! .... How?

To be precise, I was at that moment a mixture of dejection with all of its synonyms. My life's wheel came to a halt. I was squarely destined for gloom!

I retraced where I could have backslidden only to be confronted with the stupid memories of that regrettable act at club Ozone's gents, with the stranger. I needed no explanation for the cause of my strange predicament. That stranger was the source of both my infection and my pregnancy. It was like being infected with the virus and made pregnant in a dreamland! Surely, sometimes you can wake up to realize you're no longer having strange dreams but actually living those strange dreams in real life!

All my life, being infected with hiv had been the least of my expectations. I used to read in newspapers and magazines of ordeals of persons infected with the virus, however, I didn't imagine even in my wildest dreams that one day I would narrate to the world this strange testimony, me being infected with the virus. I have been caught flat-footed!

I wished I had a second chance to do everything right. What if I just walked home that evening never stepping inside club Ozone? What if I had the company of my girlfriends? Out of stupidity, I ended up contracting the aids causing virus and equally became pregnant.

My only payer is that my child will never ask me the whereabouts of his dad because I too do not know. No one knows for sure. This is surely the most ugly, unfulfilling and ill-omened journey towards parenthood. Being pregnant but unable to tell the man responsible is like knowing the truth you know nothing about!

We often look for things beyond our control yet ignore the little things that matter most in life. When faced with such calamities, we often look for avenues of passing blame to others, sometimes longing to crucify them for our own faults and blunders.

I know I made a grave mistake on that fateful day. Anyway, what happened had to happen. It's called fate. I won't dwell on that irreversible slip-up. However, I believe there are other ladies out there who may have suffered similar fate; unknowingly infected with hiv by other men known or unknown to them. My encouragement is, don't hide in the dark. Come out and seek for help. There is plenty available to seekers.

Let's share our stories, however painful they may sound to help keep our other sisters safe from immoral and vengeful men; men who pride in taking advantage of any of our sexual weaknesses. *Real men date sober women, they don't take advantage of drunken ladies.*

And to any night club-thirst sister, if you must go to any night club at night, have the company of a close friend, colleague, family or relative. Keep yourself safe from suffering similar fate. Your life is your responsibility, take proper charge of it".

The Double Accident

Anne's miserable ordeal

An accident is an accident

African Proverb

After Elizabeth had concluded her narration, Anne, the third lady and the fourth person took to the stage.

And without any hesitation, she began.

"Christmas was nearing so I wanted to replenish a few house supplies from the only local supermarket store located four kilometers away. It was a cloudy and windy afternoon that Sunday.

I boarded a public bus on my way to the supermarket.

Once the bus was full, the journey started off well. However, two kilometers a way, there was a sudden heavy downpour which impaired the bus driver's visibility. Two to three minutes later, the bus veered off the main road, hit some ditch and rolled several times before coming to a halt. Moments later, three passengers were declared dead, fourteen others severely wounded, and the rest registered minor injuries, I included.

There was a lady in her mid thirties who was seated next to me in the bus. The accident left her with deep body cuts and severe bleeding. She later on succumbed to her injuries. Unfortunately, at the time of the accident, both of us had not placed our safety belts on. We ended up tightly embracing each other the moment the vehicle veered off the road and rolled. Unluckily, it was that terrifying life-saving embrace that led to both of us coming into direct contact with each other's blood, from our openly bleeding body cuts. Unluckily still, this other lady was hiv-positive and sadly, that was how I ended up contracting the deadly aids causing virus. It was like a double accident that Sunday afternoon!

At the time of the accident, Faith, that lady as I came to know of her name later on, had neither time nor energy to disclose to me she was hiv-positive. I too, never suspected she could have been infected with the virus. Even the nurses who attended to me at Eden's general hospital after the accident never had time to test both of our blood samples and provide necessary remedy since the other lady had been directly taken to hospital's morgue.

Five months later, I had the heartbreaking revelation that I had been infected with the aids causing virus. But how? For the past ten years, I had stayed solo with zero active sex life. I had not slept with anyone in those ten years, save for the usual teenage wannabe-dad and mum-like experiences. I did establish beyond any reasonable doubt that the grisly road accident was the source of my infection. It was shocking!

How could I be infected with the virus from a road accident? I sometimes still wonder!

I have since then undergone several counseling sessions. With candor, I now do find it easy in my heart to forgive the late Faith. After all, she was no more and I equally cannot recollect how she looked like. Even if she knew she had infected me with the virus, it wasn't her intention. It was an accident and *an accident is an accident.* And why do I insist she was the cause of my infection and not the rest of the passengers? It's because we were the only two passengers seated at the back of the vehicle. During the time of the accident, we ended up tightly embracing each other for more than ten minutes and in the process, got directly exposed to each other's blood, oozing out of each of our body cuts and wounds.

Sometimes certain strange things happen that we can't explain. More often, most of us end up becoming victims of other peoples' unfortunate circumstances. However, I have come to learn that God has a reason for letting certain unexplainably strange things to happen in our lives. We may at times find ourselves in bizarre situations that want to stop our life's wheels from moving on and want to give up. Nonetheless, the problems we encounter today may either bring us down or catapult us to the next higher levels, depending on how we react to them. It is however, very unfortunate that most people fail to see how God wants to use some challenges for the good of their lives.

Sometimes life's obstacles and challenges may knock us down, time and time again. We've got to learn to push forward in such dark moments, when a majority would readily quit. We simply have to refuse to quit. The dark moments in life are usually temporary. They may last for some minutes, a few days, a few months, or even for some years, but eventually, they will subside and disappear.

During that dark period, there is an anonymous avowal which I came across. It has been my consolation all along. I clearly couldn't understand why I ended up becoming a victim of another's strange circumstance. In fact, I printed the copy of that statement and it's beautifully hanging on my sitting room's wall.

It reads

'God has a prefect reason for allowing certain things to happen in our lives. We may never understand his wisdom but we simply have to trust in his will. Life is full of challenges; it can be very stressful and uncomfortable, but it is vastly better than the alternative which is nothing. Sometimes what is best for us is not what we could often have the opportunity to choose. So, it is better to accept and live life for all that it is worth'.

When traveling via public service vehicles, always take as much necessary precaution as you possibly can such as having your safety belt on. But most importantly, do your best each and every moment whilst leaving the rest in God's hand. At times, we may fail to fathom his ways, but He has continued to assure us that His ways never fail.

Let's all lend a hand in the war against aids" She closed her narration and took to her seat.

Thinking Of Committing Suicide?

A Suicide's checklist

Remember, the wages of sin is death

A Biblical Statement

Committing suicide has never resolved any issue. Almost everyone you meet has encountered some form of disappointment, but some people end up living a thereafter life of misery out of such disappointments. They take an aimless saunter down the path of life blindfolded. Truth is sometimes our wheels may require a little adjustment or re-alignment to get back on the right track and direction.

When all seem lost and perhaps the next and only visible option is to cut off your existence through committing suicide, then that is the time to go through the below suicide's checklist.

- The biblical Judas committed suicide because he had betrayed and handed over the son of God, The Almighty, to be killed by mere human mortals. Have you betrayed Jesus to warrant committing suicide?

- Remember the proverbial 'time heals all wounds'. No matter how hurting it seems and feels, give it some time. No matter what sort of difficulties or how painful the experience is, your wound will definitely heal, in the fullness of time.

- Face your fears. Committing suicide brands you cowardice. Do not be afraid to confront issues that life has strewn along your path. Face them head on and learn the relevant lessons, where necessary.

- Live your life. Forget what other people might be thinking or saying behind your back. Your life and all that you do while here is your sole responsibility. Everyone is never perfect, and so are you.

- Joy always comes in the morning, but you must first pass through a dark night to experience that joy. Even gold is refined through fire. Exercise patience and perseverance. Remember, whatsoever is lovely has some pain or difficulty attached to it.

- Be realistic. Don't cry forever when sad moments come knocking. Yes, never hold your tears if it is really painful. However, learn and plan to move on quickly. No matter how dark moment may seem, you must learn to quickly get over it.

- Did you give it your all? If no, then keep on trying. But if you feel like you gave it your all then don't worry. You will always live to fight for another day. Sometimes what we desire might not be the best things for us.

- Committing suicide leaves issues unresolved. It is like running away from a responsibility that life has bestowed upon you.

- As a Christian, I have a strong conviction that God will never gives us challenges that we cannot overcome. He will never give you a challenge beyond your measure. Sometimes God may take us through certain painful moments in order to bring us back in harmony with him.

- *'Things are never as bad as they seem'*.... Robin Sharma. Things that cause us lots of pain, heartaches and sorrows are the same ones that prepare us for success in life.

- Some people claim that the biblical Samson opted to commit suicide after betrayal by his lovely wife Delilah. However, the bible records that at the time of his death, Samson killed more Philistines than he had killed during his lifetime. His death therefore, had a divine purpose and plan from God.

- God has not and will never give up on you. Life is a journey of struggles, with unending ups and downs. Sometimes you are happy and other times you are sad. You must keep on keeping on. Quitters never win.

- All human lives are interconnected. We all depend on each other. Ending your life means leaving millions of people who are interconnected to you hanging, without support. Ending your life means ending other million lives silently.

- What will you ever tell God on the Judgment day? That you mortgaged your mind and allowed confusion to prevail upon you? That you had thought life had lost its real meaning.........? Think beyond such lame lines. God never created you to commit suicide. You can do better than that.

- Have you considered the reaction of those who genuinely love you? Your family, friends and relatives? No matter what, there are people who will never abandon you. Their love for you cannot be traded for anything. Don't disappoint them. They will always stand with you, no matter what comes your way.

- *'A problem shared is half solved'*…Anonymous. Did you share your problem and no one came to your rescue? Did you really exhaustively share your problem?

- Do you trust in God? With a stone and a sling David killed the mighty and dreaded Goliath. He achieved this invaluable feat because he had faith and trust in God. You too posses what it takes to overcome your Goliath.

- Life goes on and the best gifts in life are hidden in the next day. Fight to claim your precious gift that tomorrow holds for you. Just hold on.

Think beyond suicide and walk an extra mile. The world will always be jam-packed with both seen and unseen turbulences. Be courageous, persistent and focused. This life is not a desert for you to wander about in any direction. Be decisive, set your goals and begin your journey. With prayers and trust in God, you will achieve your dreams. Avoid the rope. Stay safe and enjoy life.

Strange Beliefs & Misconceptions About Sex and Hiv/Aids

Six misleading beliefs and misconceptions about sex and hiv/aids

Then you will know the truth, and the truth will set you free

John 8: 32

Having Sex with a virgin will cure anyone infected with hiv/aids

This is equivalent to robbery with violence! It is an illegal act which may lead to arrest, possible conviction to life imprisonment, or even possibly death sentence.

If anyone is hiv-positive, goes ahead and enjoys unprotected sex with a virgin, the only guarantee is an infection to that innocent victim, the virgin. But this is only in case the virgin is hiv-negative.

Therefore, the least an hiv-positive person can do is to refrain from having unprotected sex with anyone to limit chances of transmitting the virus to others, or limit chances of being re-infected with the virus from other hiv-positive partners.

Once infected with the virus, you are death bound

The world's health trends are fast changing. Today, cancer has dislodged hiv/aids as the number one killer disease.

Still, the power of antiretroviral drugs has revolutionized the health sector and brought back life to many ailing and nearly dying hiv-positive patients. If infected, it isn't the end of the road. Just take the prescribed drugs and hung on. Tomorrow is a beautiful day patiently awaiting you And who knows? Maybe a cure maybe least found when no one least expects, tomorrow.

Infected adults who have sex with minors end up getting healed of the virus

Having sex with a minor is an offense before any court of law anywhere in the world. An infected adult who goes forth and performs unprotected sex with a minor will most definitely end up infecting the minor with the virus, and also getting arrested.

No one has ever come out publicly to declare being healed of the virus out of having sex with a minor. Don't be the hero! You might end up with a re-infection, or spending the rest of your life behind bars.

Having un-protected sex is sweeter, fresher and much more fulfilling than having sex with condoms on

Any successful and fulfilling satisfaction during sex is achieved when the parties involved eventfully attain orgasm. And having sex with condoms on doesn't stop or delay any party from reaching orgasm.

No research has established that use of condoms may stop any partner from reaching orgasm. Instead, having unprotected sex with a doubtful partner, may expose one to contracting the aids causing virus.

Prostitution is a lucrative and well-paying career

From recent research, it is established that prostitution is the leading cause of hiv/aids infection, especially in Africa. Yes, money out of prostitution may seem easy and probably appear lucrative, but the negative consequences of prostitution may be life threatening, especially when unprotected sex is exercised.

You are considered cursed if infected with the hiv/aids

As a Christian, I believe Jesus Christ died and was painfully, nailed on the cross to take away all of our sins. Therefore, curses no longer exist, especially to those who believe in Jesus Christ.

Facing Life's Obstacles

Understanding reasons why God may allow certain obstacles a long your way

Life is full of challenges. It is often stressful and uncomfortable. But it is vastly better than the alternative which is nothing

Anonymous

Life is not always 100% fun. Sometimes, certain strange challenges may pop out of the oblivion and unremittingly confront you. The problems you encounter today may either bring you down or turn out to be your blessings - depending on how you choose to react to them.

It is however, unfortunate how most people fail to recognize how God intends to use some challenges to better their lives. Facing challenges in life require an activation of faith within. God has a reason for permitting certain things to occur in our lives. And as anonymously noted, *we may never understand His wisdom but we simply have to trust in His will.*

There are four major reasons why God may allow difficulties along anyone's path.

- To scrutinize and rectify you.
- To give you a sense of bearing.
- To protect you.
- To bring out the best in you.

Difficulties as a tool for scrutiny and rectification

Your true potential or worth in life can sometimes be unmasked once you go through an adversity. Passing through any difficulty will hand you an honest inward evaluation of who you truly are.

A more specific example on how to approach pain and suffering is well documented in the bible. In the book of (*James 1:2-4*) the bible gives sureties that; we should consider ourselves fortunate when all forms of trials come our way. That, when our faith wins over such trials then the result is a renewed ability within us to be tolerant. That when we uphold the endurance all the way without failing, then we will be made perfect and complete, lacking nothing.

The bible also reminds us of the story of one righteous man in the name of job. That God permitted Satan to pose tribulations in Job's life just to test his unrelenting faith in God. However, in the end, Job overcame all those painful trials and temptations, and the final reward was a double portion of what he originally owned. If Job hadn't gone through that dark period, then perhaps his status quo, in terms of faith and wealth, would have remained the same, all through his life.

Difficulties and the sense of bearing

Problems or challenges you go through may provide you with the only opportunity for self reflection. They may be the only road-block on your reckless speed along the smooth road of life. They will therefore, hand you an opportunity to make a stop and possibly effect the necessary and relevant adjustments as you proceed with your journey through life.

The biblical book of (*Proverbs 3:5-8*), reminds us to put our trust in God and never to try to depend on what we think we know.

That when we let God be the everything in all we do, then He will always show us the right way.

Tribulations as a means of protection

There is an old age aphorism that *sometimes a problem may be a bigger blessing in disguise…. more so if it has an attachment of success in the aftermath.* The biblical book of *Genesis 37:12-36* tells the amazing story of Joseph. That when he was young, Joseph was almost killed by his blood related brothers, but was lucky to have been sold off by the same brothers as a slave to some Ishmaelites who were passing by. This story goes on to account how later on, God protected Joseph and made him find favor in the eyes of Potiphar; a King's officer - (*Genesis 39:1-6*). Potiphar was pleased with Joseph and took him as his personal servant. He then later on put him in charge of his house and everything he owned.

Joseph continued to find favor in the eyes of the Lord and was later on, made Governor over the whole of Egypt. After several years, Joseph miraculously re-surfaced and reminded his brothers of their past evil plot to kill him and instead greedily agreeing to sell him off as a salve …. And that through all those their weird plans, God had kept him safe and had even propelled him to greatness. It is recorded in the bible that *Joseph said to his brothers, "Please come near to me." So they came near. Then he said: "I am Joseph your brother, whom you sold into Egypt. But now, do not therefore be grieved or angry with yourselves because you sold me here; for God sent me before you to preserve life. For these two years the famine has been in the land, and there are still five years in which there will be neither plowing nor harvesting. And God sent me before you to preserve posterity for you in the earth, and to save your lives by a great deliverance. So now it was not you who sent me here, but God; and He has made me a father to Pharaoh, and lord of all his house, and a ruler throughout all the land of Egypt......(Genesis 45: 4-8 NKJV).*

God allowed Joseph to face the humiliation of being sold off to strangers. He protected him all through those strange and dark moments and later on, used him to safeguard the lives of his evil-minded brothers together with many other people who were faced by starvation, after famine had visited their country.

Problems may bring out the best in you

When we respond to problems accordingly, we grow and end up building positive characters. We should learn to celebrate when difficulties come our way, because they help us exercise the virtue of humility and patience.

Our character is who we really are and we need to keep building it. Borrowing from the same biblical story of Joseph illustrated above, had he not been sold off by his brothers, then perhaps he would have remained a herdsman all his life. However God protected him and used the evil plot of being sold off to strangers, to bring out the best in him.

God is always at work in our lives. We may never understand or even recognize it. Always surrender your plans and wishes to him because he remains the Alpha and the Omega. He knows what is perfectly good for your life. Whatever challenge may come your way, you should be ready to take it in stride.

Always Look Around

I once had no food to eat, until I met a man who had no teeth!

I once had no good shoes to wear, until I met a man who had no feet!

I once had no nice shirt to wear, until I met a man who had no arms!

I once had no money, until I met a dead beggar on a busy street!

Anonymous

When your life is on a downhill and you seem to be totally defeated, don't ever give up. Out there, someone else has it even worse. When you look around, you'll be glad yours isn't that worse! Your life could only seem like an endless curse only if you shut yourself in your own world, refusing to look around.

Always Look Around

Author's Note

The four painful stories herein are fables. Incidences, names, places and characters used herein, either are the product of the author's imagination or are fictitiously arranged. Any similarity to persons living or dead, events, or locales is entirely coincidental.

HIV – Human Immunodeficiency Virus.

AIDS – Acquired Immune Deficiency Syndrome.

Cover Image Credit: Courtesy of piaxabay.com